Happy Together

a single mother by choice double donation story

Written by Julie Marie

Illustrated by Ashley Lucas

This book is dedicated to Ashley Lucas. Thank you for bringing Happy Together to life through the wonderful illustrations.

ISBN-13: 9798988355908

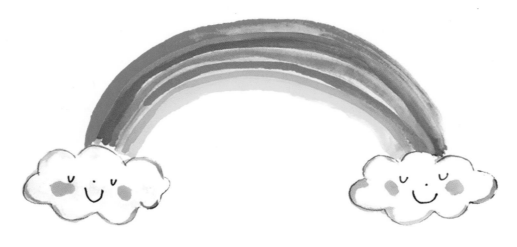

Happy Together

a single mother by choice double donation story

Written by Julie Marie

Illustrated by Ashley Lucas

The sun was shining bright
And the sky was blue above,

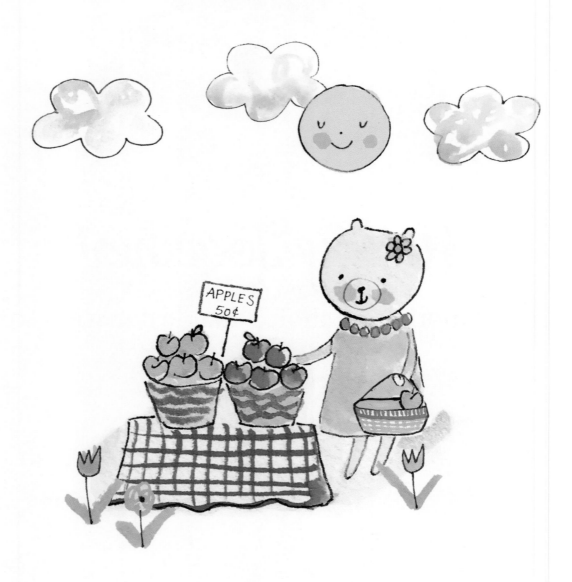

Mommy had a happy life full of friends
And family with lots and lots of love.

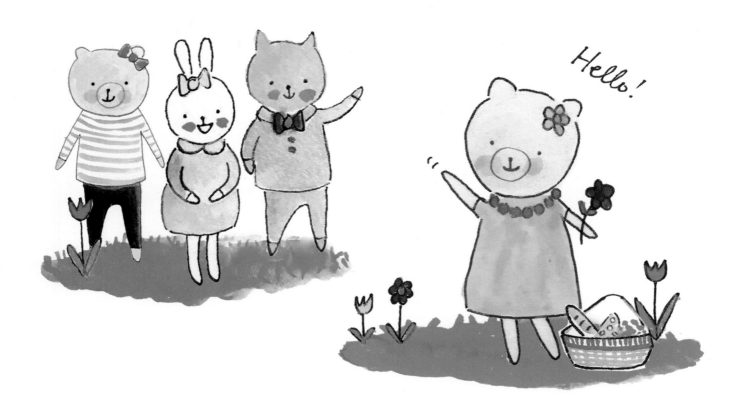

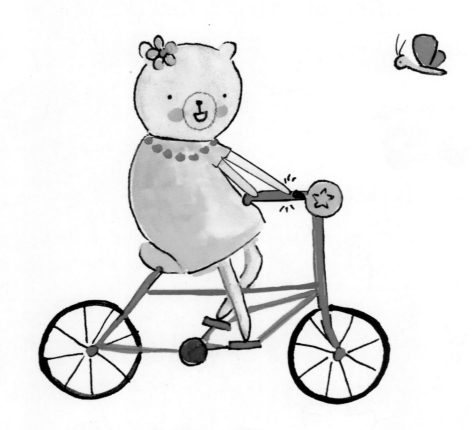

Mommy went on many adventures
Laughing, smiling and having fun,

I had a great future ahead and wanted
To share it with a special little someone.

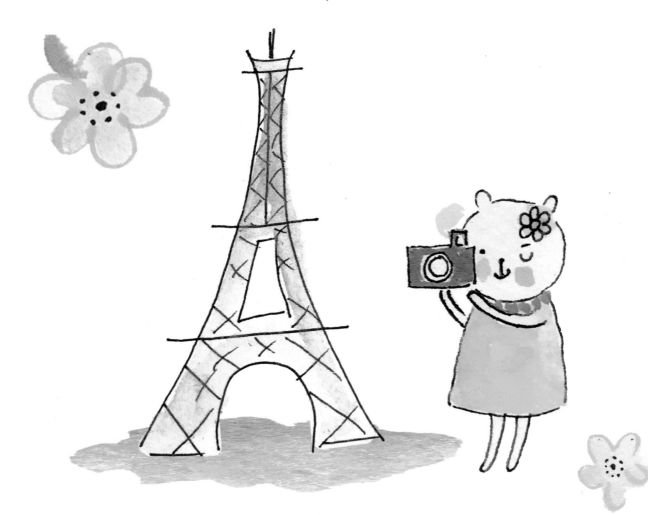

Wish

Deep within my heart
Mommy had a special wish
More than anything I wanted to have a baby
To love, hug and kiss!

For some parents

It's easy to have a baby

And for some parents

It's not.

For your Mommy

I knew my journey to have you

Would take a lot.

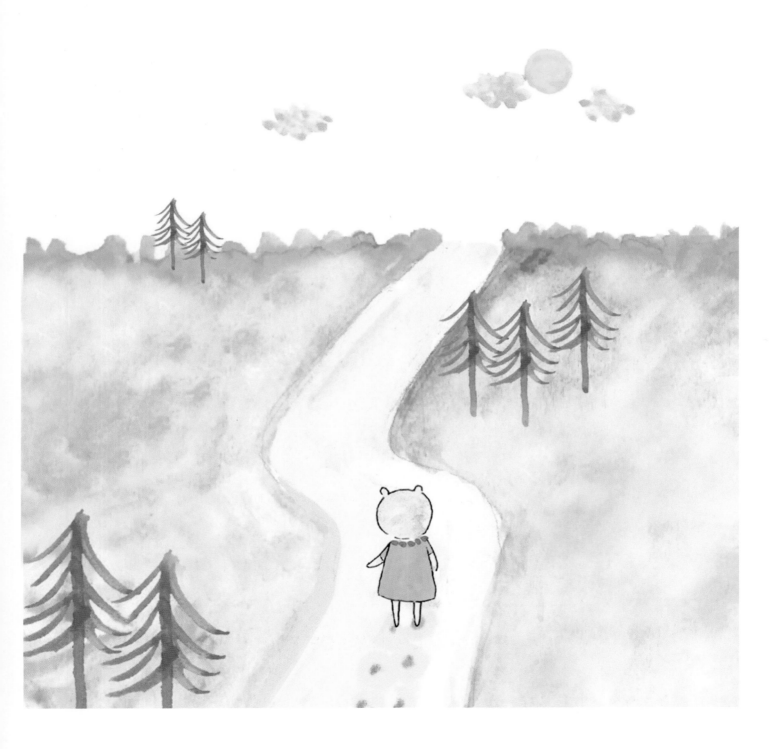

To make a baby
It takes a seed from a male
And an egg from a female.
Mommy didn't have a seed and my eggs
Weren't working and couldn't make a baby.

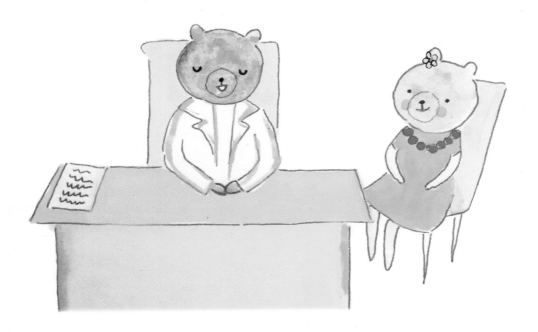

Mommy went to a doctor
And talked about my plan
To have a baby I would need the help
Of a very special lady and man.

The special man and lady are donors
And they gave the seed and egg.

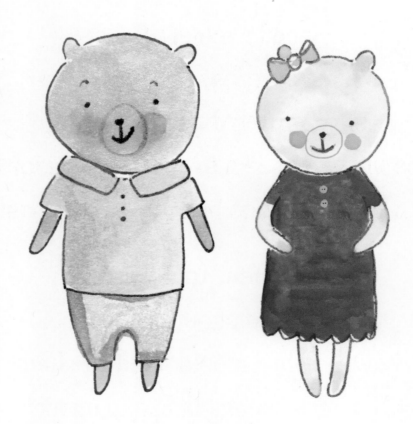

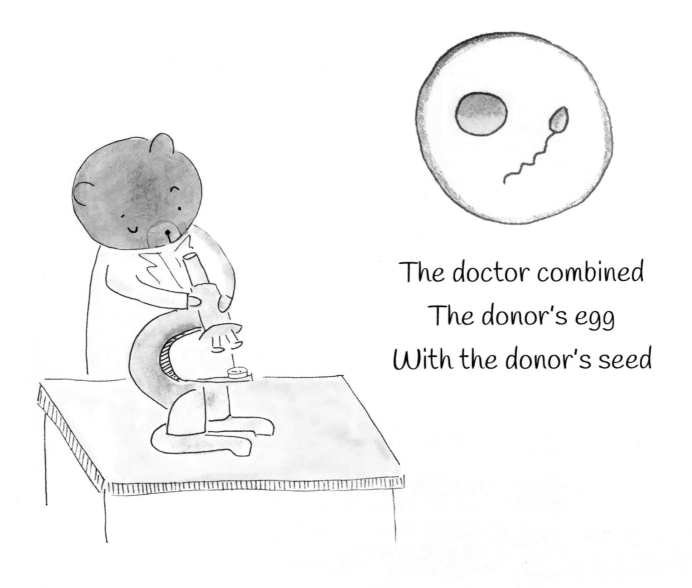

The doctor combined
The donor's egg
With the donor's seed

Then he transferred it into Mommy's tummy
And it turned out to be exactly what I would need!

Once again, the sun was shining bright one day
The sky was blue above
That's when Mommy received the best news
I was pregnant with you
And my heart was full of love!

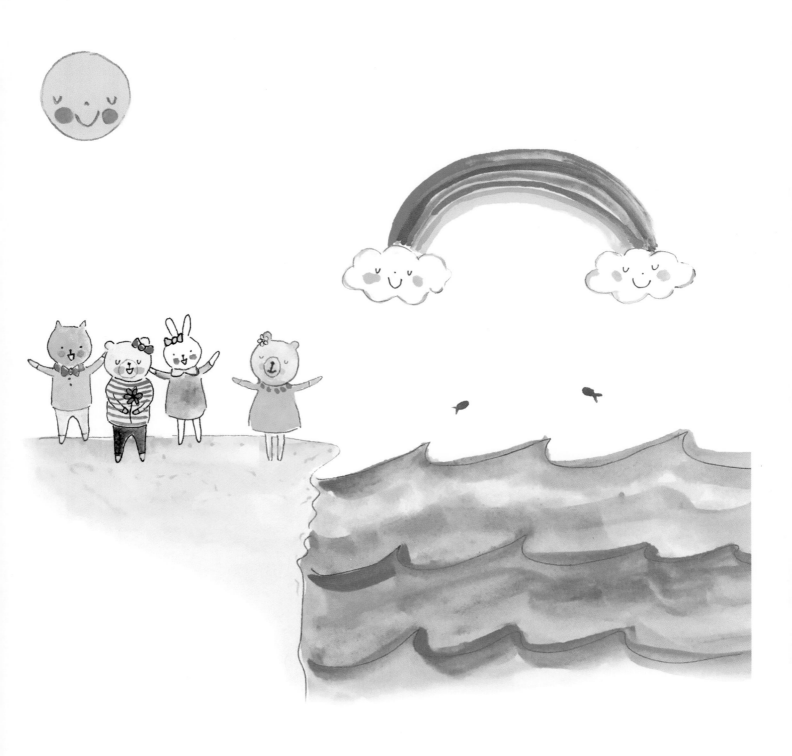

As the months passed by

Bigger and bigger Mommy's tummy grew,

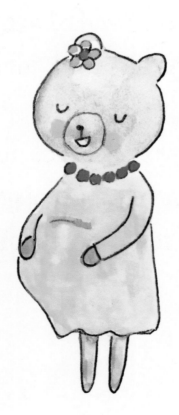

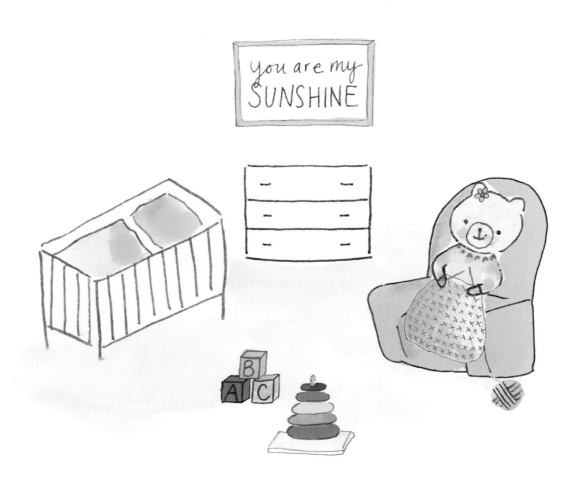

I cheerfully prepared for your arrival
Mommy was so excited to meet you!

The day you were born
My dream of having a child came true,

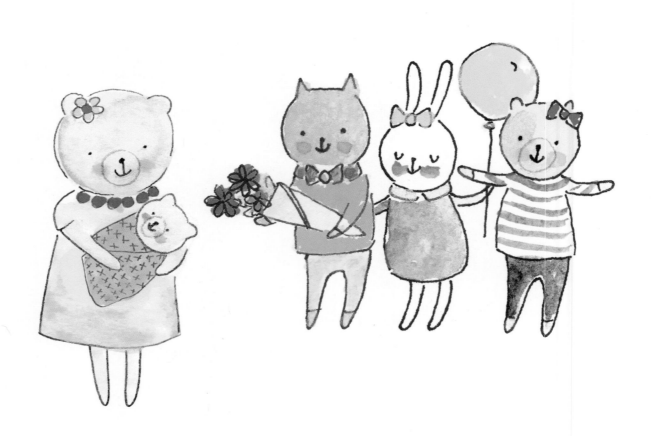

Mommy was beyond grateful
To finally be able to love, hug and kiss you!

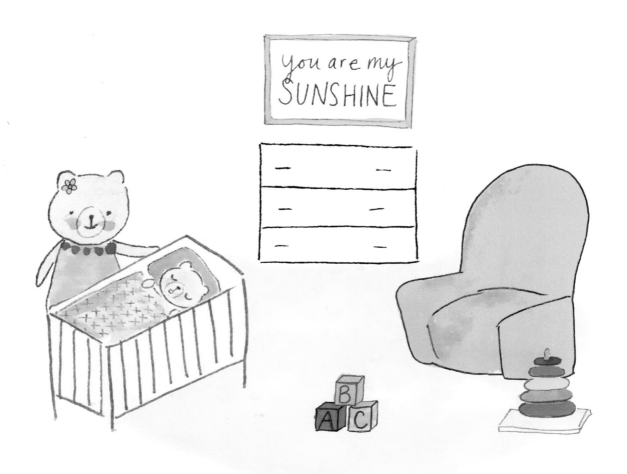

Happy together, we are a family

Mommy's love for you is beyond measure,

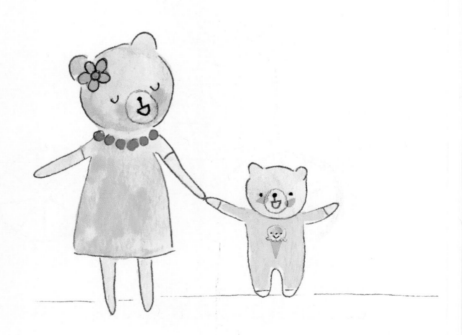

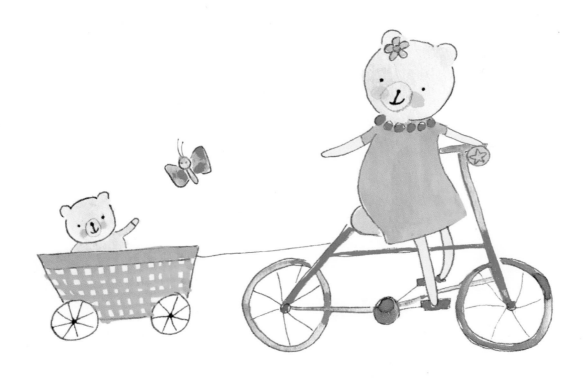

We laugh, smile and have fun

Making memories we will always treasure!

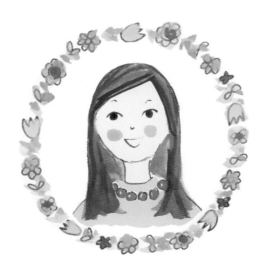

JULIE MARIE

I am an infertility advocate
and mother through IVF.

It is my hope that Happy Together
will provide a heartwarming,
family building story for parents
to read with their child
sharing just how much they were
wished for and loved.